Bolster Your Spirit

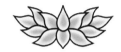

By Mana Iluna
and
Kathy Triplett

D1504861

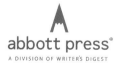

abbott press®

A DIVISION OF WRITER'S DIGEST

BOLSTER YOUR SPIRIT
First Edition 2011

Abbott Press books may be ordered through booksellers or by contacting:

Abbott Press
1663 Liberty Drive
Bloomington, IN 47403
www.abbottpress.com
Phone: 1-866-697-5310

ISBN: 978-1-4582-0123-2 (sc)

Printed in the United States of America

Abbott Press rev. date: 12/5/2011

Table of Contents

Foreword

With life on the go and stress on the rise, this book is the perfect antidote. It is time to return to a balanced life where effort is supported by rest and rejuvenation.

These beautiful postures allow your body to open effortlessly, your mind to experience stillness, and your Spirit to nourish both. These pages hold many possibilities for finding your way to harmony. The gentle postures are the keys to entering a new space where you are able to embrace and replenish your self and to Bolster Your Spirit.

Notes from the Authors

Recommended Yoga Props

The following yoga props are recommended for the postures used in Bolster Your Spirit. Yoga props including bolsters are available online. You can also substitute firm pillows for bolsters and foam pads.

     1-2 Bolsters, 1 Belt, 1 Blanket, 2-4 Foam Pads

The Heart Center

There are many references to the Heart Center in Bolster Your Spirit. The Heart Center is the master energy center of the body. It is helpful to focus on a simple flame of white light deep within the center of the chest. Concentrate on the flame of white light in the Heart Center to quiet your mind and bring a feeling of peace and love into your mind and body.

Please Note: Welcome your body into each pose, and stay as long as your body and mind remain comfortable. Even with a program as gentle as this, a qualified healthcare professional should be consulted. If you are pregnant, your midwife or ob/gyn should be consulted before you begin this or any other fitness program. As with any exercise program, if at any time you experience discomfort, stop immediately and consult your physician or healthcare professional. The authors are not responsible for any injuries that may result from attempting the poses herein.

With Gratitude

Gratitude is akin to and a necessary part of love in its purest form.

With that concept in our hearts, we express our deepest, heartfelt gratitude to The Mother, whose inspiring thoughts grace this book, and to the Sri Aurobindo Ashram for the permission to publish them from the book Rays of Light (available at www.yogacenters.com).

To Aadil Palkhivala and Savitri, our gratitude is boundless for creating Yoga Centers, the home of Purna Yoga, and Purna Yoga itself. Together, Savitri and Aadil have molded and guided our lives in wondrous ways over the years and have given their invaluable expertise to shape the contents of this book.

Our gratitude flows to Arya Pretlow, who generously agreed to allow her lovely images of yoga on the bolster to grace these pages.

To all, we say thank you, thank you, thank you.

Meditation Posture - I

The Pose:

- Sit on the side of the bolster near the edge.
- Fold the legs on the floor in front of the body.
- Lift the lower abdomen.
- Keep the spine vertical and erect.
- Move the kidneys gently toward the chest.
- Rest the hands on the thighs, palms up.
- Relax the elbows toward the floor.
- Lift the sternum while lowering the shoulder blades.
- Keep the chin parallel to the floor.
- Relax the neck, throat and shoulders.
- Rest the eyes and mind on the flame of white light glowing in the Heart Center.

The Benefits:

- Allows one to quiet the body and focus the mind in the Heart Center.

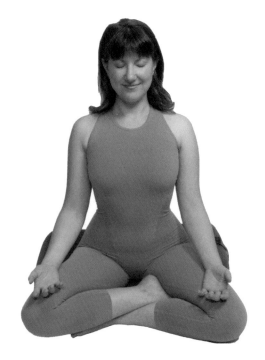

Meditation Posture - II

The Pose:

- Sit on the end of the bolster near the edge.
- Fold the legs on the floor in front of the body.
- Lift the lower abdomen.
- Keep the spine vertical and erect.
- Move the kidneys gently toward the chest.
- Rest the hands on the thighs, palms up.
- Relax the elbows toward the floor.
- Lift the sternum while lowering the shoulder blades.
- Keep the chin parallel to the floor.
- Relax the neck, throat and shoulders.
- Rest the eyes and mind on the flame of white light glowing in the Heart Center.

The Benefits:

- Allows one to quiet the body and focus the mind in the Heart Center.

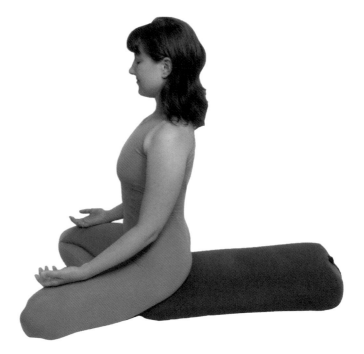

Baddha Konasana - Supported

 "It is in silence that the soul best expresses itself." —————————————

The Pose:

- Sit on the side or end of the bolster (for people with more open hips, a foam pad can be used to catch the buttocks in back, with the sitting bones on the floor).
- Bring the soles of the feet together.
- Hold the ankles.
- Lift the lower abdomen.
- Keep the spine vertical.
- Move the kidneys toward the chest.
- Keep the chin parallel to the floor.
- Press the soles of the feet together to move the knees apart.
- With open or closed eyes, keep the inner gaze at the Heart Center.

The Benefits:

- Sitting on a bolster allows the hips to open more easily and keeps the back from rounding.
- Opens the groin muscles.
- Strengthens the spine.
- Circulates energy through the pelvis.
- Eases menstrual discomfort.

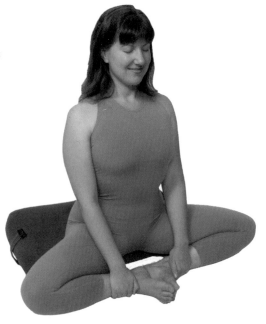

Virasana - I

 "To express Harmony, of all things Simplicity is the best."———————————

The Pose:

- Sit on the front end of the bolster.
- Bring both feet back to rest next to the bolster.
- If the tops of the feet or ankles are uncomfortable, place a rolled blanket under each ankle.
- If the knees are uncomfortable, place one or two foam pads under the buttocks.
- If there is sharp pain in the knees, do not do this pose.
- Move the knees directly forward from the hips.
- Lift the lower abdomen.
- Keep the spine vertical.
- Lift the sternum as the shoulder blades move down.
- Keep the chin parallel to the floor.
- Rest the hands on the thighs, palms up.

This is a good meditation posture when crossed legs become uncomfortable.

The Benefits:

- Keeps the knee joints flexible.
- Allows the hip muscles to release.
- Strengthens the spine.
- Stretches the tops of the feet, keeping them flexible.

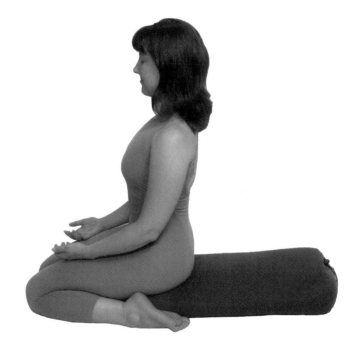

Virasana - II

The Pose:

- Kneel on the bolster.
- Place the folded blanket to touch the back of the knees between the thighs and calves, and sit down, with the toes off the bolster.
- There must be no sharp pain in the knees. If there is add extra blankets.
- Lift the lower abdomen.
- Keep the spine vertical.
- Lift the sternum as the shoulder blades move down.
- Keep the chin parallel to the floor.
- Rest the hands on the thighs, palms up.

This is a good meditation posture when crossed legs become uncomfortable.

The Benefits:

- Helps open the knee joints.
- Releases the hips.

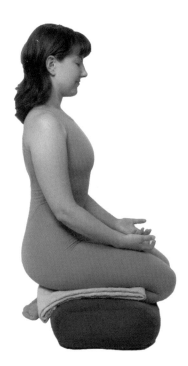

Virasana - III

 "It is only in quietness and peace that one can know what is the best thing to do." ————————

The Pose:

- Sit on the side of the bolster with the knees forward and the lower legs under the bolster.
- Bring the big toes together, with the lower legs and the feet on a blanket if necessary for comfort.
- It is acceptable for the heels to move apart even though the big toes are together.
- There must be no sharp pain. If there is, add extra blankets.
- Lift the lower abdomen.
- Keep the spine vertical.
- Lift the sternum as the shoulder blades move down.
- Keep the chin parallel to the floor.
- Rest the hands on the thighs, palms up.

This is a good meditation posture when crossed legs become uncomfortable.

The Benefits:

- Opens compressed knee joints.
- Keeps the knee joints flexible.
- Allows the hip muscles to release.
- Strengthens the spine.
- Stretches the tops of the feet, keeping them flexible.

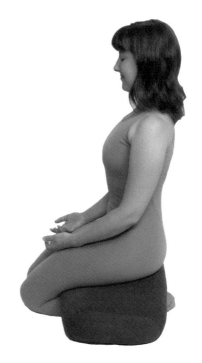

Eka Pada Supta Virasana

 "Sweetness adds its smiling touch to life without making a fuss."

The Pose:

- Sit 3 inches away from the bolster.
- Bring one foot back with the knee directly forward from the hip.
- The forward knee should touch the floor. If it doesn't, place another bolster under the body so that the knee releases to the floor.
- There should be no sharp pain in the knee. If there is, place another bolster on top of the bolster so there is less pull on the quadriceps and knee.
- There should be no low-back discomfort. If there is, place a foam pad under the buttocks.
- Bend the other leg, with the foot on the floor next to the inner thigh.
- Lie down on the bolster with your head on the foam pad (if the neck feels uncomfortable, place a foam pad or blanket under the head).
- Bring the arms away from the body to open the armpits, palms up.
- Alternate legs, so both sides receive the benefit of the pose.

The Benefits:

- Relaxes the diaphragm.
- Opens the lungs.
- Lengthens the abdominal muscles.
- Aids digestion.

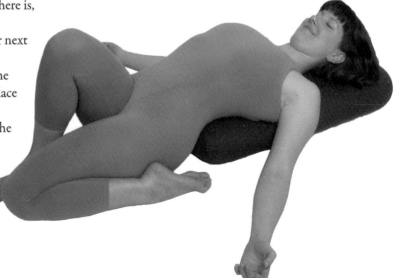

Supta Virasana

 "It is the heart that has wings, not the head."

The Pose:

- Place two bolsters with the top one 6 to 10 inches behind the bottom bolster.
- Sit on the bottom bolster.
- Place both knees forward, and bring the feet next to the bolster.
- Keep the knees directly forward from the hips.
- Rest the hands on the feet (or outward as shown, palms up).
- Place three foam pads in front of the bottom bolster under the buttocks, then lie back on both bolsters for additional knee comfort.
- There must be no sharp pain in the knees.

The Benefits:

- Relaxes the diaphragm.
- Opens the lungs.
- Lengthens the abdominal muscles.
- Aids digestion even better than Eka Pada Supta Virasana.

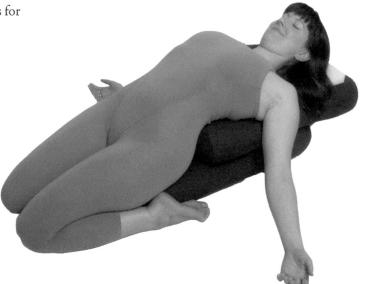

Bhujangasana

 "The hopes of today are the realizations of tomorrow."

The Pose:

Not recommended for individuals with chronic low-back problems.

- Lie on the bolster with the tops of the thighs at the bottom of the bolster.
- Place the hands under the shoulders with the elbows touching the body.
- Tighten the buttocks, and move the tailbone toward the heels.
- Move the shoulder blades toward the buttocks.
- Inhale, press the hands into the floor, and push the upper body off the bolster. (Raise the upper body off the bolster only as far as it feels comfortable for the low back.)
- Move the sternum forward.
- Reach into the toes — stay for three breaths.
- Spread the feet hip-width apart to further release the lower back if necessary.

The Benefits:

- Maintains flexibility of the spine.
- Moves the spine counter to its usual forward bend.
- Opens the Heart Center.
- Strengthens the arms.
- Strengthens the back muscles.

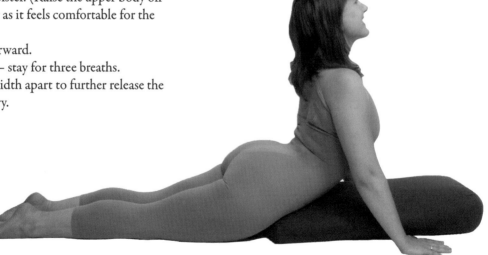

Adho Mukha Shvanasana

The Pose:

It is best not to do this pose during the menstrual cycle.
- Place the hands beside the bolster a little wider than the shoulders, fingers wide.
- Place the top of the forehead on the bolster and/or foam pads as the feet move back 3 to 4 feet from the bolster. Spread the feet hip-distance apart.
- Lift the buttocks toward the ceiling.
- Extend the sides of the body toward the sitting bones as the heels descend toward the floor.
- Relax as much as possible, with enough weight on the head to help support the body along with the shoulders, hands and arms.

The Benefits:

- Lengthens and releases the spine.
- Gentle inversion allows release of abdominal organs from gravitational pull, allowing circulation and stimulation in this area.
- Gently stretches the hamstring muscles.
- Opens and strengthens the shoulders and arms.
- Stretches the Achilles tendon and calf muscles.
- Supporting the head allows one to stay longer in the pose, for enhanced benefits.

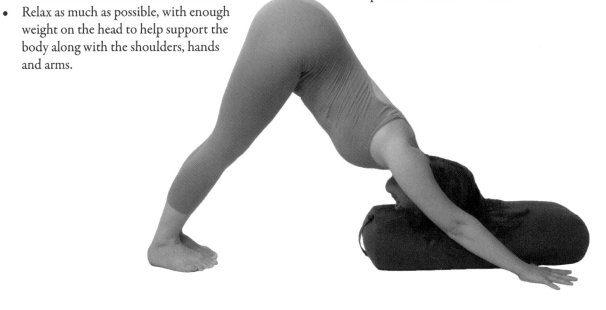

Supta Baddha Konasana

 "To conquer the difficulties there is more power in a smile than in a sigh." _____

The Pose:

- Sit about 3 inches in front of the bolster.
- Bring the soles of the feet together comfortably close to the body.
- Place the belt loop around the back at the sacral area, under the toes, and over the thighs and adjust firmly.
- Support the knees by placing blankets or foam pads under them. (There must be no pulling or discomfort in the groin area.)
- Lie down, and move the tailbone toward the heels. (If the low back feels uncomfortable, place a blanket or foam pad under the buttocks.)
- Place the head on one or more foam pads for comfort.
- Bring the arms away from the body to open the armpits, palms up.
- Move the shoulders toward the floor.

The Benefits:

- Opens the Heart Center.
- Allows the body to feel open, supported and deeply relaxed.
- Aids the circulation of energy in the pelvis.
- Gently stretches the abdominal muscles.
- Relaxes the shoulder and neck area.
- Especially useful during menses.
- The longer one stays in this pose, the greater the benefit.

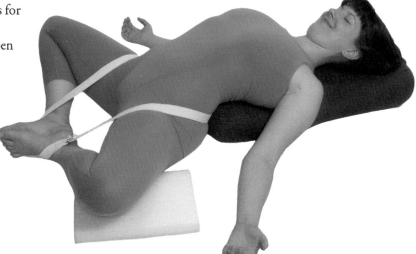

Back Bend - On Cross Bolsters

 "A drop of practice is better than an ocean of theories, advises and good resolutions." ———————

The Pose:

- Cross two bolsters.
- Lie on the length of the top bolster.
- Bring the legs together with the belt around the mid-thighs, soles of the feet on the wall.
- Variation 1: Don't use the belt, and just allow the legs and feet to relax apart.
- Variation 2: Place the back of the neck at the curved end of the top bolster to support the neck and relax the head back.
- Bring the arms above the shoulders.
- If it is more comfortable, stretch both arms to the sides. (If the shoulders can't find a comfortable place, hold each elbow and place the arms above the head.)

The Benefits:

- Gently stretches the front body, quadriceps, and upper and lower abdomen.
- Opens the chest and shoulders, making breathing easier.
- Relaxes the neck and throat.
- Supports the spine, allowing the spinal muscles to release.
- Curves the spine in the opposite direction from the usual rounding forward.
- The belt keeps the legs together while they relax.

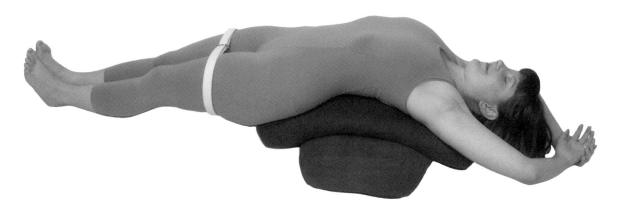

Setu Bandha Sarvangasana - I

 "Always remember that on the happiness you give will depend the happiness you get." _____

The Pose:

- Align two bolsters lengthwise.
- Sit on the bolster to place the belt around the mid-thighs.
- Lie down.
- Slide back until the tops of the shoulders rest on the floor.
- Bring the arms away from the body to open the armpits, palms up.
- Keep the legs straight.
- Relax the neck, throat and shoulders.
- Rest the eyes and mind on the flame of white light glowing in the Heart Center.

The Benefits:

- Opens the chest and diaphragm.
- Gently removes the forward bend of the upper back.
- Aids the circulatory system.
- Releases the gravitational pull on the abdominal organs and legs.
- The belt keeps the legs together while they relax.

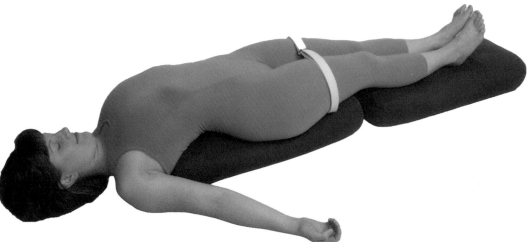

Setu Bandha Sarvangasana - II

 *"Your soul blossoms to the Light as a flower opens to the sun."*_____

The Pose:

- Cross two bolsters.
- Sit on the bottom end of the top bolster.
- Place the belt around the mid-thighs.
- Lie down and slide back until the head and shoulders rest comfortably, heels on the wall. (If the low back feels uncomfortable, place two foam pads at the bottom end of the top bolster, as shown.)
- Move the tailbone toward the heels.
- Relax the neck, throat and jaw.
- Bring the arms above the shoulders with the right hand in the left hand.
- If more comfortable, stretch both arms to the sides. (If the shoulders can't find a comfortable place, hold each elbow and place the arms above the head.)

The Benefits:

- Opens the chest and the Heart Center.
- Gently stretches the chest, rib cage and back muscles.
- Reverses the usual forward curve of the spine.
- Increases the flow of oxygen into the lungs.
- The belt keeps the legs together while they relax.

Viparita Karani - I

 "To conquer a desire brings more joy than to satisfy it." _____

The Pose:

Avoid this pose during menses or if you have high blood pressure or a heart or eye condition.
- Place the bolster 2 inches from and parallel to the wall.
- Lie on the bolster with the buttocks touching the wall. (If the hamstrings are tight, move the bolster farther from the wall and move the buttocks a comfortable distance from the wall.)
- Rest the upper back, head and shoulders on the floor.
- Place the belt around the mid-thigh.
- Bring the arms out, palms up.
- Draw the shoulder blades toward the wall.

The Benefits:

- Releases the hips and low back.
- Gentle cardiac stimulation.
- Opens the chest.
- Gently removes the forward bend of the upper back.
- Stimulates and energizes the kidneys.
- Reverses gravitational pull.
- Reverses the blood flow from the legs and feet.
- The belt keeps the legs together while they relax.

Viparita Karani - II

 "Try to be happy - immediately you will be closer to the Light." _____

The Pose:

Avoid this pose if you have high blood pressure or a heart or eye condition.

- Cross two bolsters.
- Place the lower bolster 1½ inches (or farther for comfort) from the wall and parallel to it.
- Lie on the length of the top bolster with the legs up the wall.
- Support the neck at the curve of the top bolster.
- Place the belt around the legs at mid-thigh.
- Bring the arms out to the side, palms up.

The Benefits:

- Keeps the spine flexible.
- Opens the chest.
- Gentle cardiac stimulation.
- Reverses gravitational pull.
- Reverses the blood flow from the legs and feet.
- The belt keeps the legs together while they relax.

Heart Opening - I

 "The nobility of a being is measured by its capacity of gratitude."

The Pose:

- Lie over the side of the bolster.
- Bring the shoulders slightly off the bolster until the arms can rest comfortably out to the side, palms up (shoulders should not touch the floor).
- Move the shoulder blades toward the buttocks.
- Keep the buttocks on the floor.
- Rest the head on the floor.
- If the low back is uncomfortable, place one or two foam pads under the buttocks.
- If the neck is uncomfortable, place one or two foam pads under the head.
- Relax the legs (if preferred, a belt can be used at mid-thigh).

The Benefits:

- Opens the chest.
- Opens and relaxes the diaphragm.
- Creates flexibility in the back.
- Reverses the forward curve in the spine.

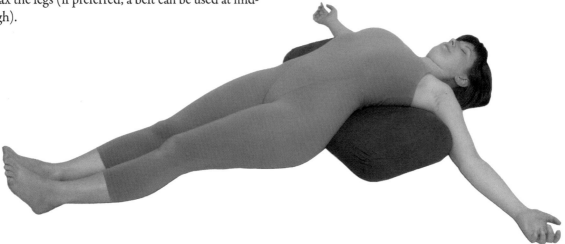

Heart Opening - II

 "Yoga is commensurate with all life." —

The Pose:

- Lie over the side of the bolster.
- Rest the neck at the curve of the back side of the bolster. (It is important for the neck to rest in the bolster's curve to keep the neck curve supported.)
- Rest the Heart Center at about the middle of the bolster, depending on the length of the torso.
- Hold each arm above the elbow, and place the arms above the head.
- Reach elbows upward from the shoulders.
- Relax the legs, or a belt can be used around mid-thigh.

The Benefits:

- Opens the chest.
- Creates flexibility in the upper back.
- Reverses the forward curve in the upper spine.
- Opens the shoulders and stretches the shoulder joints.

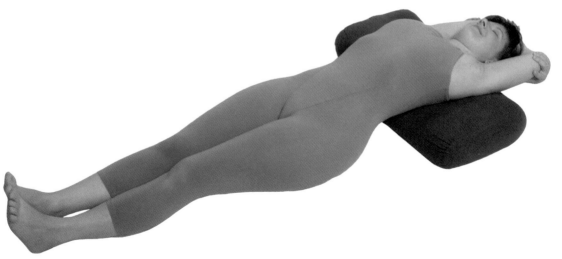

Janu Sirsasana

 "If you want peace upon earth first establish peace in your heart."

The Pose:

Avoid this pose if you have back issues or low blood pressure.
- Bend one knee, bringing it to the side even with the hip. (If the bent knee is off the floor, place a blanket or a foam pad under the knee.)
- Place the sole of the bent-leg foot against the side of the thigh.
- Straighten the other leg.
- Place the bolster on the straight leg.
- Move the navel in line with the straight leg.
- Lengthen the front of the body, placing the forehead on one or more foam pads.
- Holding the belt in each hand, place the belt around the bottom of the straight-leg foot.
- Alternate legs.

The Benefits:

- Quiets the mind and restores the body.
- Supports the low back while maintaining flexibility in the spine.
- Rests the abdominal muscles.
- Gently opens the hip.
- Gently stretches the muscles on each side of the spine.

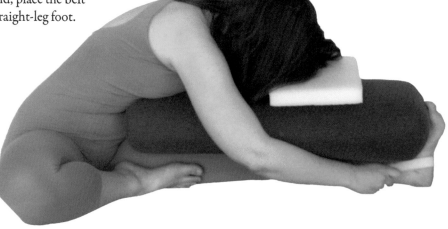

Pregnancy Resting Pose - 1

 "They always speak of the rights of love but love's only right is the right of self-giving." ⸻

The Pose:

- Lie with one side on the floor.
- Place the bolster between the bent legs. (A large pillow can also be used.)
- Place the head on the bolster.
- Straighten the lower arm or bend it slightly above the head.
- Rest the upper arm on the bolster.

The Benefits:

- Releases the low back muscles.
- Keeps the low back comfortable and able to rest.
- Keeps the spine relaxed while at rest.
- Supports the abdomen on the floor.

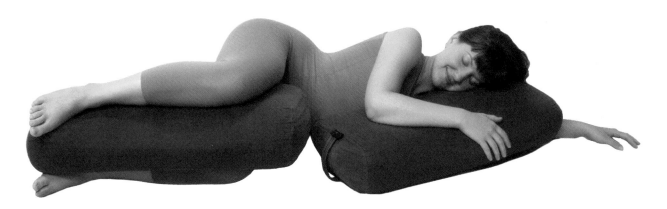

Pregnancy Resting Pose - II

 "The world is deafened by useless words."

The Pose:

- Lie with one side on the floor.
- Place the length of the bolster in front of the lower leg.
- Place the bent upper leg on the bolster.
- Place the head on the second bolster. (A blanket or pillow can be placed under the head. The head should be even with the spine.)
- Relax both of the shoulders and the arms.

The Benefits:

- Releases the low back muscles.
- Rests the hips comfortably.
- Keeps the spine relaxed while at rest.
- Supports the head and neck to aid relaxation.

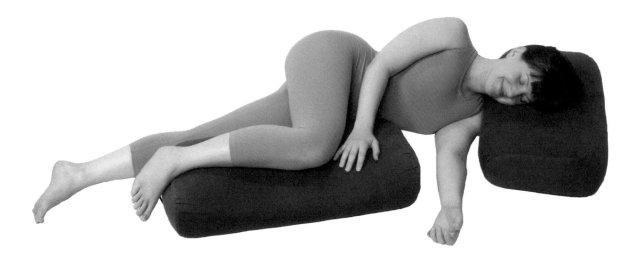

Side Stretch

 "If you can always smile at life, life also will always smile at you." _____

The Pose:

- Lie with your side on the bolster.
- Rest the rib cage at the center of the bolster.
- Bring both arms overhead, palms together.
- Rest the head on the lower arm.
- Bend the knees for comfort and balance.
- Relax the neck and throat.
- Alternate sides.

The Benefits:

- Opens the rib cage.
- Stretches the muscles between the ribs.
- Opens the shoulder joints.
- Increases oxygen flow into the body.

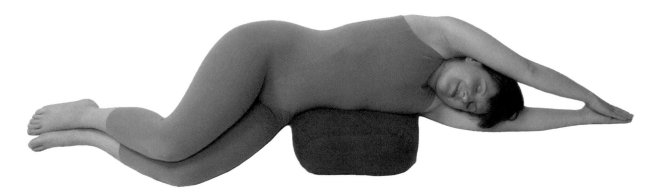

Balasana - Child's Pose

 "To know is good, to live is better, to be, that is perfect."

The Pose:

Avoid this pose during pregnancy.
- Sit on the heels, toes together.
- Open the knees as wide as comfortably possible.
- Bring the bolster between the knees and close to the body.
- Keep the buttocks on the heels as you lie across the bolster.
- There are three ways to place the head and arms:
  1. Rest the arms in front of the shoulders (as shown). For comfort, alternate turning the head from one side to the other.
  2. Place the hands on top of each other to rest the forehead on the hands.
  3. Bring the hands near the feet to spread the shoulder blades apart.

The Benefits:

- Highly beneficial for low-back discomfort or pain.
- Opens the hip joints.
- Keeps the knees flexible.

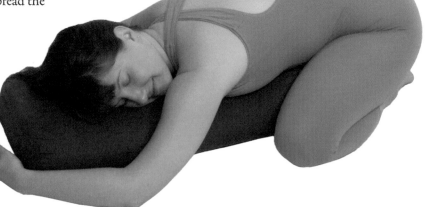

Tummy Rest

 "Liberation: the disappearance of the ego." ——————————————————————

The Pose:

Avoid this pose during pregnancy.
- Cross the bolsters.
- Lie lengthwise on the top bolster.
- Rest the chin on the end of the bolster.
- Roll the shoulders forward and down toward the floor.
- Rest the arms, palms facing the ceiling.
- Relax the legs completely.

The Benefits:

- Relaxes the neck and shoulders.
- Presses the abdomen, allowing the abdominal muscles to relax.
- Releases and relaxes the back.
- Releases the spinal muscles from holding the spine erect.
- Opens the back side of the rib cage.

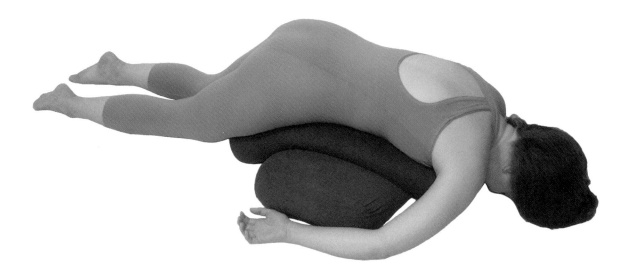

Pranayama Posture

 "Self-mastery is the greatest conquest, it is the basis of all enduring happiness." ———————

The Pose:

- Lie down, placing the entire rib cage on the bottom of the bolster.
- Place the head on a foam pad, with the forehead slightly higher than the chin.
- Bring the arms away from the body to open the armpits, palms up.
- Relax the shoulders toward the floor.
- Relax the feet and legs completely.
- If there is low-back discomfort, tilt the pelvis so the tailbone moves away from the head, and/or bend the knees and place a rolled blanket or bolster under the knees.

The Benefits:

- Gently opens the chest and rib cage to allow the breath to flow more freely into the lungs.
- Relaxes the whole body, while allowing more oxygen to enter the body.
- Relaxes tension in the diaphragm.

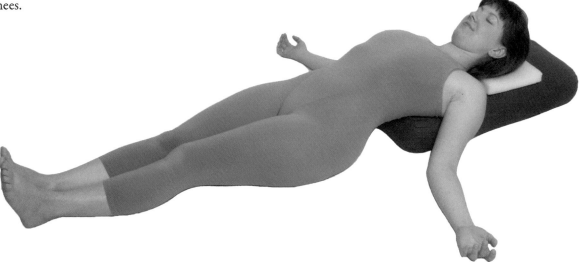

Shavasana - I

 "To know how to wait is to put Time on your side."

The Pose:

- Lie on the floor with the knees supported on the bolster.
- Rest the heels on the floor.
- Separate the shoulder blades slightly.
- Bring the arms away from the body to open the armpits, palms up.
- Release the shoulders toward the floor.
- If there is low-back pain, place another bolster under the knees and the lower legs.
- Rest the eyes and mind on the flame of white light glowing in the Heart Center.

The Benefits:

- Releases the low back.
- Allows the body to rest without low-back discomfort.

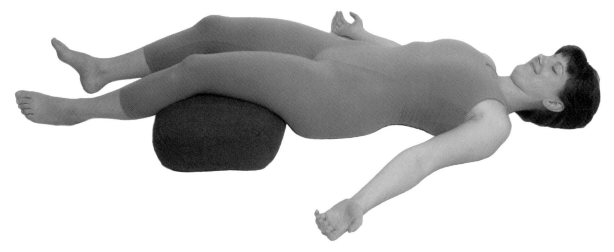

Shavasana - II

 "What is truly needed will surely come."

The Pose:

- Place the belt at mid-thigh so the legs are held comfortably together.
- Lie down, placing the legs on the bolster.
- Bring the arms away from the body to open the armpits, palms up.
- Gently separate the shoulder blades.
- Release the shoulders toward the floor.

The Benefits:

- Belt holds the legs, allowing them to be supported and fully relaxed.
- Keeps the low back comfortable while allowing the body to relax completely.
- Rest the eyes and mind on the flame of white light glowing in the Heart Center.

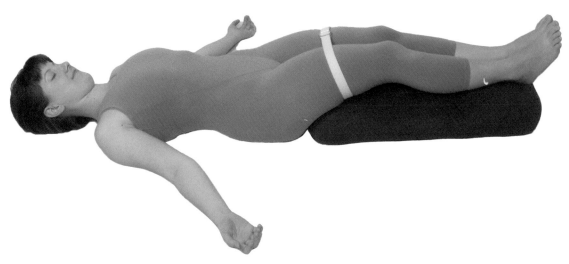

ABOUT THE MOTHER

The Mother was born in Paris on February 21, 1878. She came to India, where she met Sri Aurobindo and settled there at the age of 36. While they worked together, the Sri Aurobindo Ashram developed, and it is flourishing still in Pondicherry, South India.

Concerning her early spiritual life, she stated, "Between 11 and 13 a series of psychic and spiritual experiences revealed to me not only the existence of God but man's possibility of manifesting Him upon earth in a life divine."

To learn more about the Mother and the Sri Aurobindo Ashram, go to www.sriaurobindoashram.org.

ABOUT PURNA YOGA

Purna Yoga distills and integrates the vast aspects of yoga into an invaluable set of tools for transformation and healing. Offering wisdom and techniques for the union of the body and the mind with the spirit, Purna Yoga teaches alignment-based asana, meditation and pranayama, along with nutrition and yogic living. Purna Yoga is the art of loving yourself by living from the heart.

For information about Purna Yoga, please visit our website at www.purnayoga.com. For information about Purna Yoga Centers, please visit www.yogacenters.com.

Purna Yoga was founded by Sri Aurobindo and is expounded by Aadil Palkhivala and Savitri.

ABOUT MANA ILUNA AND KATHY TRIPLETT

Mana Iluna, MSW, is a Certified Purna Yoga™ Instructor at the 2,000-hour level, as well as an Experienced Registered Yoga Teacher with Yoga Alliance. She also teaches Purna Yoga Meditation.™ Mana has taught biweekly restorative yoga classes for twenty years at Purna Yoga Centers,™ the home of Purna Yoga.™

Kathy Triplett has used her invaluable design and technical skills to contribute to the function and beauty of this book. She teaches Purna Yoga Meditation™ and the business class in the College of Purna Yoga,™ and she is the manager of Purna Yoga Centers™ in Bellevue, WA.

ABOUT ARYA PRETLOW

Arya began practicing yoga in 1993 and started teaching in 2002. In addition to teaching yoga, she is a trained doula and a member of Pacific Association for Labor Support (PALS).

Arya is a Certified Purna Yoga™ Instructor at the 2,000-hour level, as well as an Experienced Registered Yoga Teacher with Yoga Alliance.

CPSIA information can be obtained
at www.ICGtesting.com
Printed in the USA
BVIC01n1721011013
332561BV00001B